Pocket Atlas
of
Head and Neck
MRI Anatomy

Robert B. Lufkin, M.D.
William N. Hanafee, M.D.

Department of Radiology
Medical Center
University of California
Los Angeles, California

Raven Press New York

Raven Press, 1185 Avenue of the Americas, New York, New York 10036

Made in the United States of America

Library of Congress Cataloging-in-Publication Data

Lufkin, Robert B.
  Pocket atlas of head and neck MRI anatomy.

  Includes bibliographies and index.
  1. Head—Anatomy—Atlases.   2. Neck—Anatomy—Atlases.   3. Head—Magnetic Resonance Imaging—Atlases.   4. Neck—Magnetic resonance imaging—Atlases.   5. Head—Anatomy—Handbooks, manuals, etc.   6. Neck—Anatomy—Handbooks, manuals, etc.   I. Hanafee, William N., 1926-   .   II. Title. [DNLM: 1. Head—anatomy & histology—atlases.   2. Neck—anatomy & histology—atlases.   3. Magnetic Resonance Imaging—atlases.   WE 17 L949p]
  QM535.L84   1989   611′.91′0222   88-42529
  ISBN 0-88167-498-2

The material contained in this volume was submitted as previously unpublished material, except in the instances in which credit has been given to the source from which some of the illustrative material was derived.

Great care has been taken to maintain the accuracy of the information contained in the volume. However, neither Raven Press nor the editors can be held responsible for errors or for any consequences arising from the use of the information contained herein.

9 8 7 6 5 4 3 2

Preface

This text is designed to provide a portable atlas of head and neck anatomy as seen in magnetic resonance imaging. The anatomic landmarks are displayed in axial, sagittal, and coronal MR image planes.

Most images in the text were obtained using mildly T1-weighted spin-echo sequences (Tr = 500–1000; Te = 30) in order to maximize fat/muscle contrast for maximum visualization of fascial planes, which are very valuable in head and neck anatomy.

Surface coils were used in certain areas of anatomy, where they provided significant advantages in signal to noise over standard head or body coils such as the neck and temporal bone. Images were obtained on a widely available commercial whole body iron core resistive MR instrument operating at 0.3 Tesla (FONAR B-3000M, Melville, NY).

The image plane of section and location is indicated on a labeled illustration for each view. The anatomy is labeled with numbers, which correlate with an accompanying legend for each page. For more detailed treatment of anatomy of the head and neck, the interested reader is referred to articles in the reference list.

This volume will be of interest to physicians who are interpreting MR images or are referring patients for MR studies and to fellows, residents, and medical students who are learning anatomy of the head and neck.

Contents

Neck, Larynx _____

1, internal jugular vein
2, common carotid artery
3, trachea
4, airway
5, thyroid gland
6, sternocleidomastoid
   muscle
7, esophagus

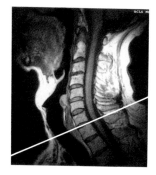

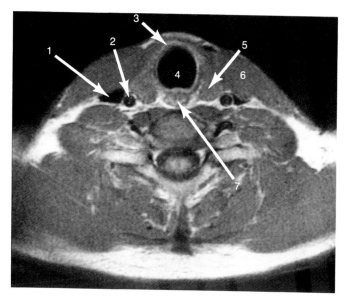

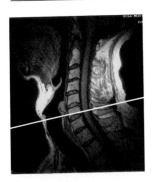

1, internal jugular vein
2, common carotid artery
3, thyroid gland
4, airway
5, cricoid cartilage
6, sternocleidomastoid
   muscle
7, postcricoid region

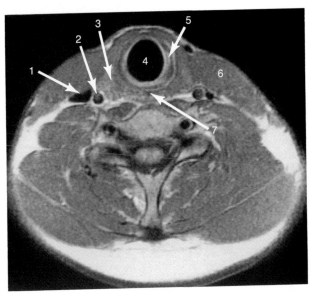

1, internal jugular vein
2, common carotid artery
3, airway
4, lamina of cricoid cartilage
5, inferior cornu of thyroid cartilage
6, sternocleidomastoid muscle

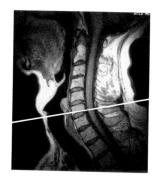

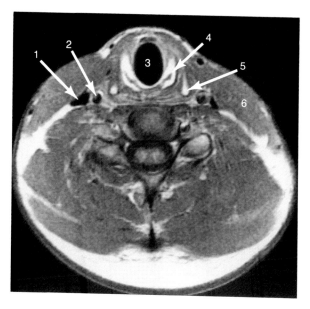

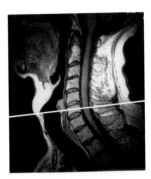

1, strap muscles
2, arytenoid cartilage
3, airway
4, anterior commissure
5, true vocal cord
6, thyroid cartilage
7, common carotid artery
8, internal jugular vein
9, sternocleidomastoid
   muscle

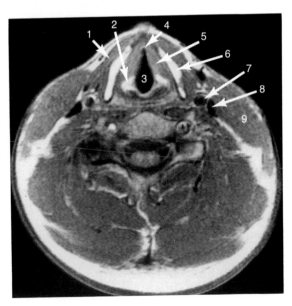

1, internal jugular vein
2, common carotid artery
3, strap muscles
4, pre-epiglottic space
5, thyroid cartilage
6, paralaryngeal space
7, airway
8, sternocleidomastoid
   muscle

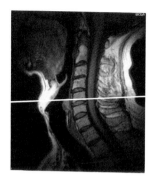

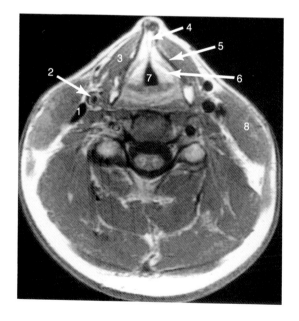

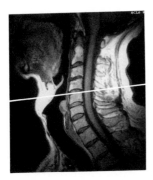

1, sternocleidomastoid
   muscle
2, thyroid cartilage
3, airway
4, aryepiglottic fold
5, piriform sinus
6, common carotid artery
7, internal jugular vein

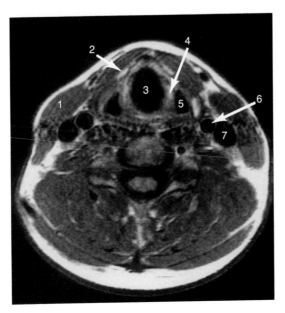

1, airway
2, strap muscles
3, pre-epiglottic space
4, epiglottis
5, submandibular gland
6, piriform sinus
7, common carotid artery
8, internal jugular vein
9, sternocleidomastoid
   muscle

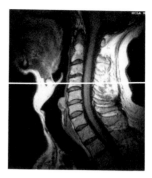

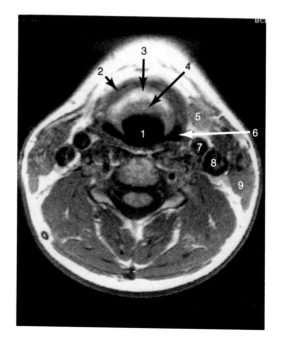

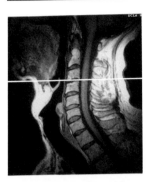

1, internal jugular vein
2, internal carotid artery
3, external carotid artery
4, submandibular gland
5, strap muscles
6, hyoid bone
7, lingual tonsil
8, free margin of epiglottis
9, sternocleidomastoid
   muscle

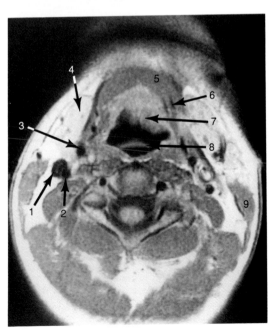

1, pre-epiglottic space
2, hyoid bone
3, free margin of epiglottis
4, arytenoid cartilage
5, cricoid cartilage
6, postcricoid region
7, trachea
8, thyroid cartilage

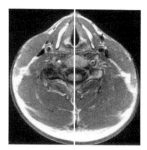

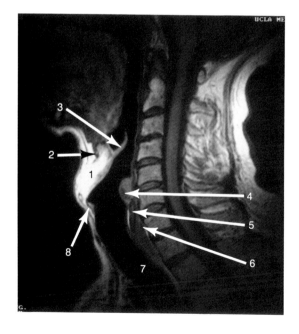

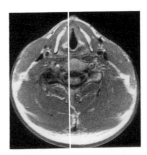

1, false vocal cords
2, hyoid bone
3, pre-epiglottic space
4, free margin of epiglottis
5, arytenoid cartilage
6, cricoid cartilage
7, postcricoid region
8, trachea
9, true vocal cords
10, laryngeal ventricle

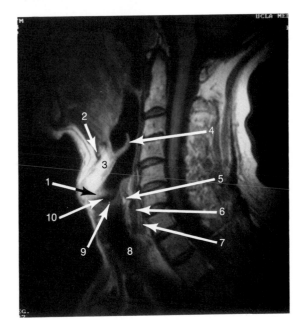

1, strap muscles
2, hyoid bone
3, pre-epiglottic space
4, free margin of epiglottis
5, paralaryngeal space
6, arytenoid cartilage
7, cricoid cartilage
8, thyroid cartilage

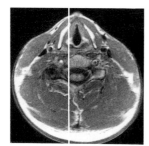

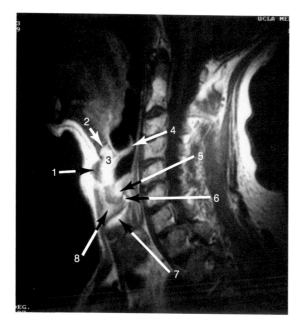

1, hyoid bone
2, paralaryngeal space
3, piriform sinus
4, thyroid cartilage

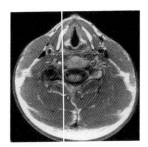

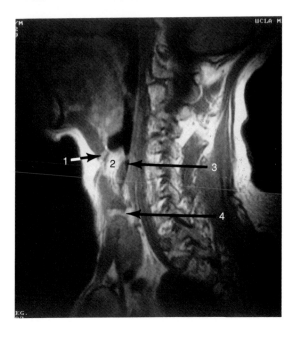

1, hyoid bone
2, vertebral artery
3, thyroid cartilage
4, strap muscles

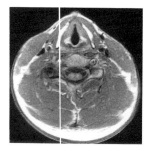

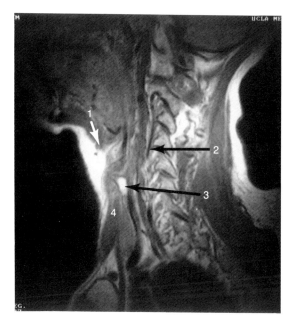

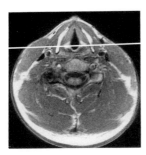

1, thyroid cartilage
2, piriform sinus
3, aryepiglottic fold
4, epiglottis
5, hyoid bone
6, arytenoid cartilage
7, cricoid cartilage
8, trachea

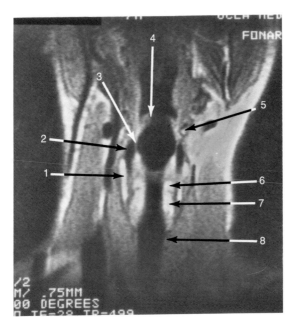

1, true vocal cords
2, paralaryngeal space
3, piriform sinus
4, hyoid bone
5, thyroid cartilage
6, cricoid cartilage

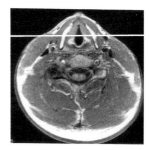

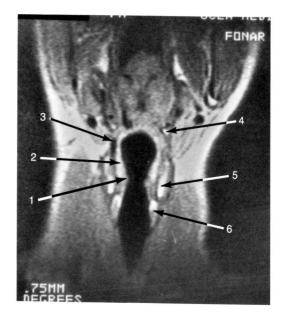

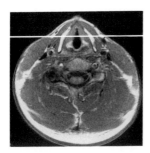

1, true vocal cords
2, paralaryngeal space
3, valleculae
4, hyoid bone
5, ventricle
6, thyroid cartilage
7, cricoid cartilage

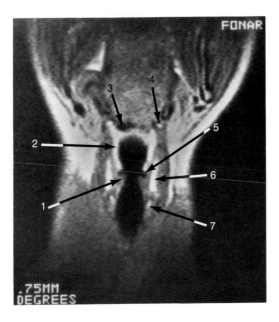

1, true vocal cords
2, paralaryngeal space
3, submandibular gland
4, pre-epiglottic space
5, hyoid bone
6, ventricle
7, thyroid cartilage

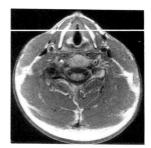

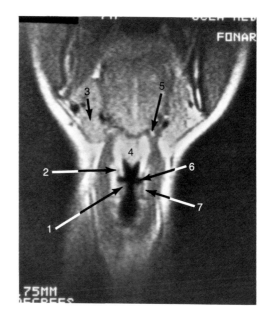

Oropharynx, Tongue ___

1, mandible
2, anterior belly of digastric muscle
3, mylohyoid muscle
4, hyoid bone
5, submandibular gland
6, vallecula
7, epiglottis
8, sternocleidomastoid muscle
9, airway

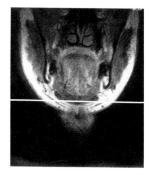

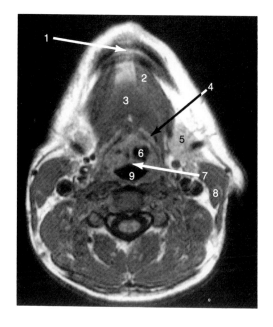

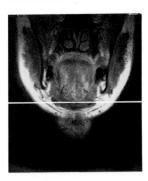

1, epiglottis
2, mandible
3, mylohyoid muscle
4, lingual septum
5, platysma muscle
6, submandibular gland
7, external carotid artery
8, sternocleidomastoid
   muscle
9, internal carotid artery
10, internal jugular vein

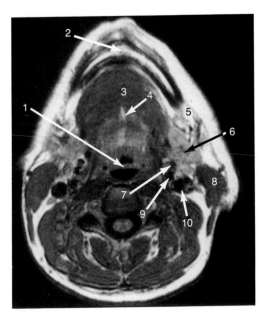

1, submandibular gland
2, lingual septum
3, mandible
4, genioglossus muscle
5, lingual artery
6, interdigitation of styloglossus and hyoglossus muscles
7, mylohyoid muscle
8, masseter muscle
9, lingual tonsil
10, sternocleidomastoid muscle

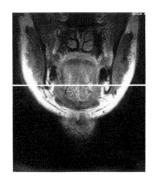

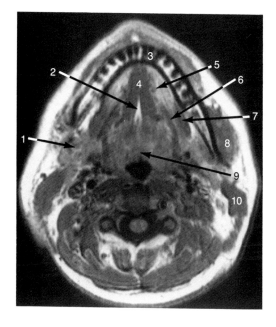

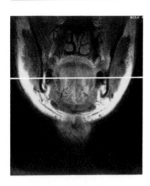

1, mandible
2, lingual artery branches
3, genioglossus muscle
4, lingual septum
5, teeth
6, superior longitudinal intrinsic tongue muscles
7, masseter muscle
8, medial pterygoid muscle
9, palatine tonsil
10, parotid gland
11, prevertebral muscle

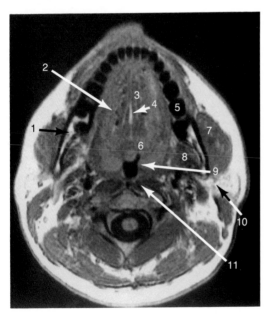

1, medial pterygoid muscle
2, masseter muscle
3, alveolar ridge of maxilla
4, mobile tongue
5, mandible
6, neurovascular canal
7, parotid gland
8, retromandibular vein
9, parapharyngeal space
10, airway

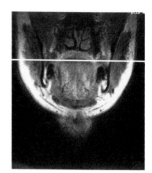

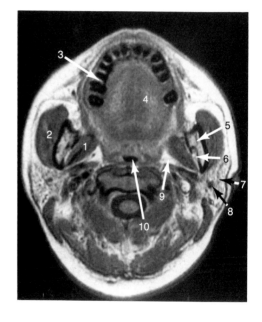

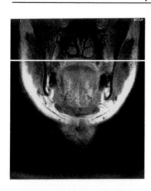

1, parapharyngeal space
2, soft palate
3, hard palate
4, maxilla
5, pterygoid plates
6, masseter muscle
7, medial pterygoid muscle
8, mandible
9, retromandibular vein
10, parotid gland
11, passavant's muscle
12, prevertebral muscles

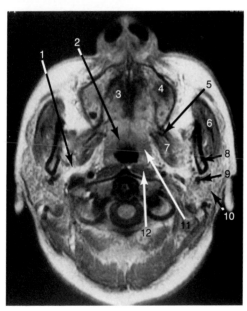

1, maxillary sinus
2, pterygopalatine fossa
3, lateral pterygoid muscle
4, medial pterygoid muscle
5, teeth
6, mandible

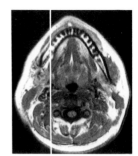

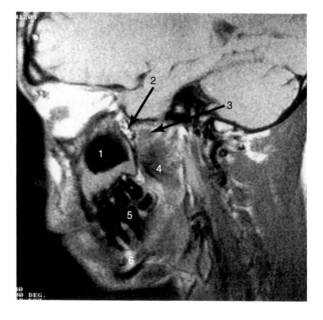

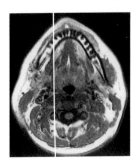

1, pterygopalatine fossa
2, maxillary sinus
3, teeth
4, mandible
5, geniohyoid muscle

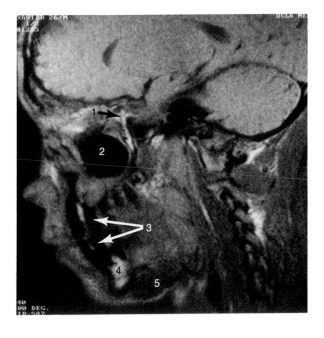

1, mandible
2, teeth
3, hard palate
4, soft palate
5, uvula
6, superior longitudinal intrinsic muscle
7, lingual artery branches
8, geniohyoid muscle
9, epiglottis

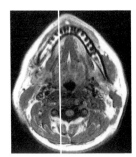

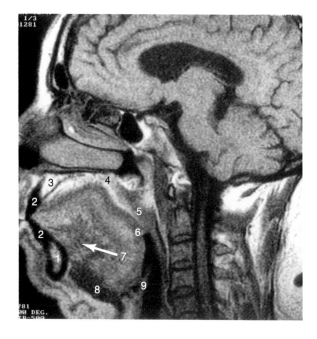

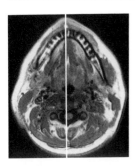

1, mandible
2, teeth
3, hard palate
4, soft palate
5, uvula
6, superior longitudinal intrinsic muscle
7, transverse intrinsic muscle
8, genioglossus muscle
9, geniohyoid muscle
10, epiglottis

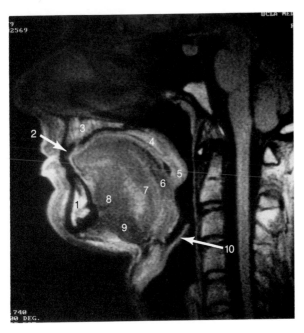

1, submandibular gland
2, sphenoid sinus
3, parapharyngeal space
4, lateral pterygoid muscle
5, medial pterygoid muscle
6, mandible
7, masseter muscle
8, palatine tonsil

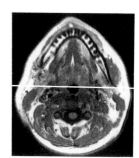

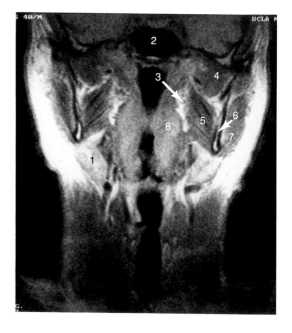

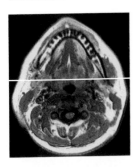

1, submandibular gland
2, lingual tonsil
3, parapharyngeal space
4, lateral pterygoid muscle
5, masseter muscle
6, mandible
7, medial pterygoid muscle
8, interdigitation of styloglossus and hyoglossus muscles
9, hyoid bone

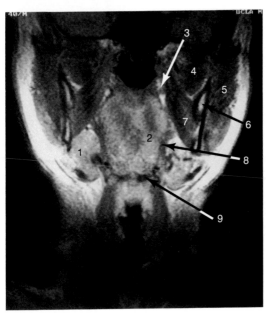

1, mylohyoid muscle
2, interdigitation of styloglossus and hyoglossus muscles
3, mobile tongue
4, genioglossus muscles
5, masseter muscle
6, mandible
7, geniohyoid muscles
8, anterior belly of digastric muscle
9, platysma muscle
10, lingual septum

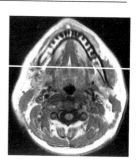

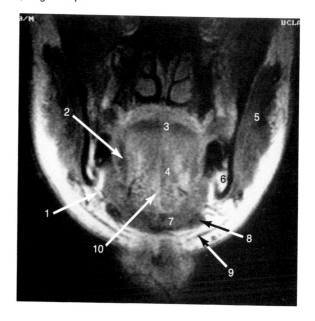

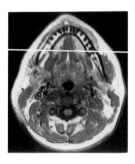

1, lingual artery
2, lingual septum
3, mobile tongue
4, genioglossus muscles
5, teeth
6, mandible
7, mylohyoid muscles
8, geniohyoid muscles
9, anterior belly of digastric muscle

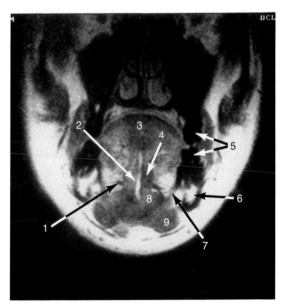

1, mobile tongue
2, lingual septum
3, teeth
4, genioglossus muscle
5, mandible
6, geniohyoid muscle
7, mylohyoid muscle
8, anterior belly of digastric
   muscle

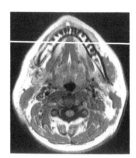

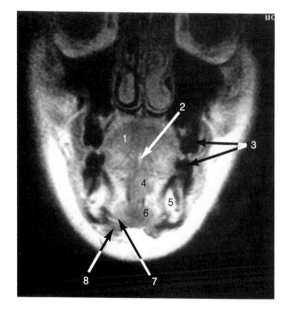

Nasopharynx, Skull Base, Sinuses _____

1, masseter muscle
2, medial pterygoid muscle
3, mobile tongue
4, maxilla
5, parapharyngeal space
6, mandible
7, retromandibular vein
8, parotid gland
9, mastoid air cells

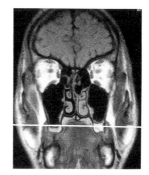

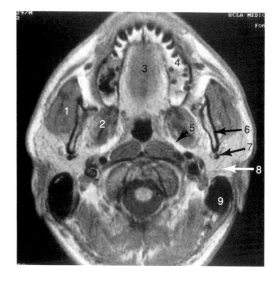

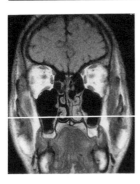

1, parapharyngeal space
2, fossa of Rosenmueller
3, levator palatini muscle
4, eustachian tube oriface
5, tensor palatini muscle
6, lateral pterygoid plate
7, medial pterygoid plate
8, nasal septum
9, inferior turbinate
10, maxillary sinus
11, coronoid of mandible
12, medial pterygoid muscle
13, lateral pterygoid muscle
14, maxillary artery branches
15, torus tubarius
16, jugular vein
17, prevertebral muscles
18, pharyngobasilar fascia

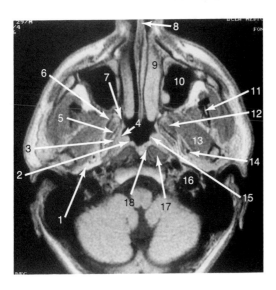

1, tensor palatini muscle
2, pharyngobasilar fascia
3, maxillary sinus
4, coronoid of mandible
5, lateral pterygoid muscle
6, condyle of mandible
7, internal carotid artery

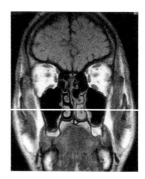

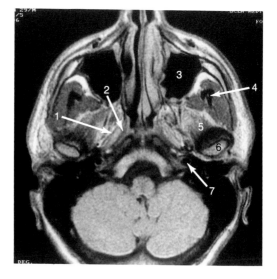

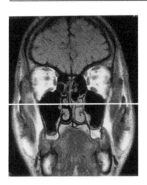

1, zygomatic arch
2, nasal septum
3, maxillary sinus
4, maxillary artery branches
5, sphenomaxillary fissure
6, mandible
7, pterygopalatine fossa
8, internal carotid artery
9, clivus

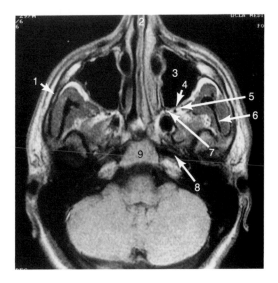

1, temporal bone
2, temporal lobe
3, nasolacrimal duct
4, orbital fat
5, maxillary sinus
6, maxillary artery branches
7, sphenoid sinus
8, internal carotid artery
9, clivus

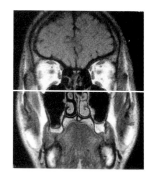

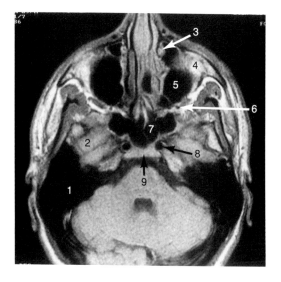

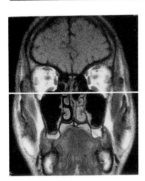

1, ethmoid sinuses
2, nasolacrimal duct
3, globe
4, orbital fat
5, inferior orbital fissure
6, sphenoid sinus
7, carotid artery

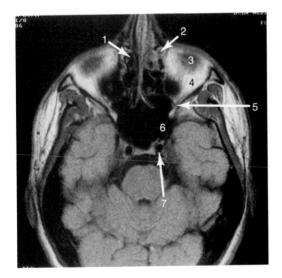

1, ethmoid sinus
2, nasolacrimal duct
3, nasal septum
4, nasal vault
5, globe
6, sphenoid sinus
7, cavernous carotid artery
8, pituitary fossa

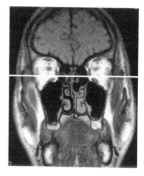

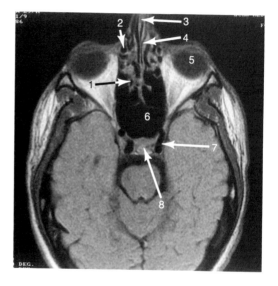

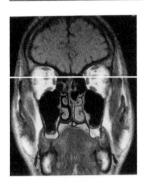

1, ethmoid sinus
2, medial rectus muscle
3, globe
4, lateral rectus muscle
5, optic nerve
6, optic chiasm
7, infundibulum

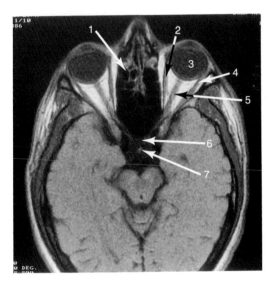

1, orbital fat
2, crista galli
3, ethmoid sinus
4, globe
5, lacrimal gland
6, superior ophthalmic vein

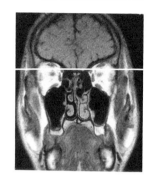

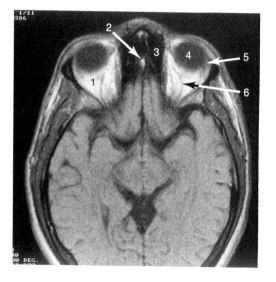

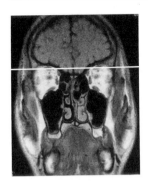

1, orbital roof
2, frontal sinus
3, frontal lobe

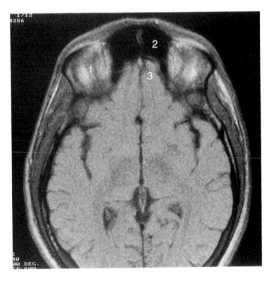

1, frontal lobe
2, frontal sinus

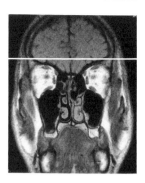

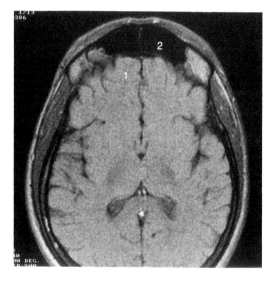

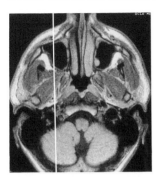

1, inferior rectus
2, globe
3, frontal sinus
4, superior rectus
5, pterygopalatine fossa
6, temporal lobe
7, foramen ovale
8, maxillary sinus
9, medial pterygoid
    muscle
10, teeth
11, mandible

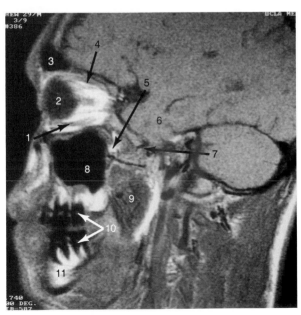

1, globe
2, frontal sinus
3, maxillary sinus
4, medial rectus
5, pterygopalatine fossa
6, foramen rotundum
7, gasserian ganglion
8, medial pterygoid
   muscle
9, teeth
10, mandible

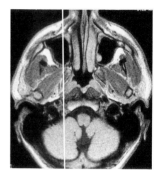

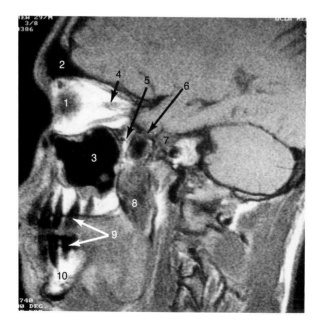

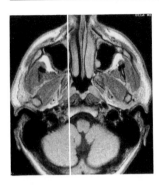

1, frontal sinus
2, maxillary sinus
3, medial rectus
4, pterygopalatine fossa
5, ophthalmic branch of V
6, trigeminal nerve
7, internal carotid artery
8, lateral pterygoid muscle
9, teeth

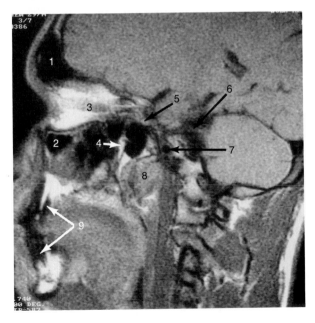

1, hard palate
2, inferior turbinate
3, frontal sinus
4, ethmoid sinus
5, sphenoid sinus
6, carotid artery

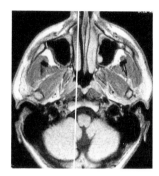

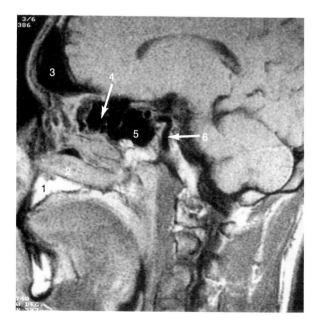

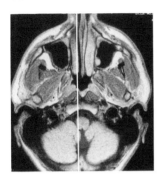

1, frontal sinus
2, ethmoid sinuses
3, inferior turbinate
4, middle turbinate
5, sphenoid sinus
6, optic nerve
7, oculomotor nerve
8, carotid artery
9, clivus

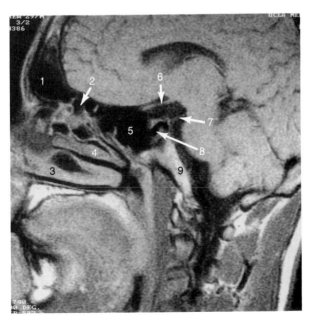

1, nasal septum
2, frontal sinus
3, crista galli
4, ethmoid sinus
5, hard palate
6, optic nerve
7, pituitary gland
8, sphenoid sinus
9, clivus
10, nasopharynx
11, oropharynx

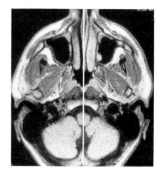

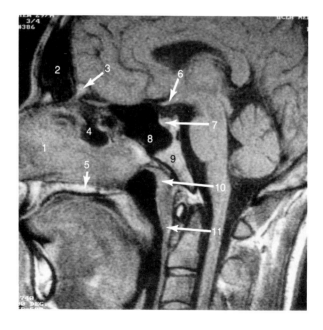

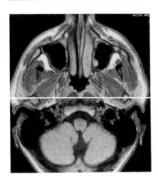

1, carotid artery
2, optic chiasm
3, infundibulum
4, pituitary gland
5, sphenoid sinus
6, gasserian ganglion
7, clivus
8, condyle
9, lateral pterygoid muscle
10, mandible
11, parapharyngeal space
12, medial pterygoid muscle
13, longus coli muscles

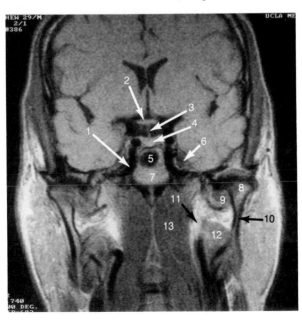

1, masseter muscle
2, mandible
3, optic nerve
4, carotid artery
5, foramen ovale
6, levator palatini muscle
7, lateral pterygoid muscle
8, parapharyngeal space
9, medial pterygoid muscle
10, pharynx

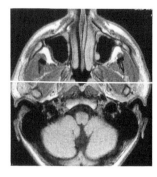

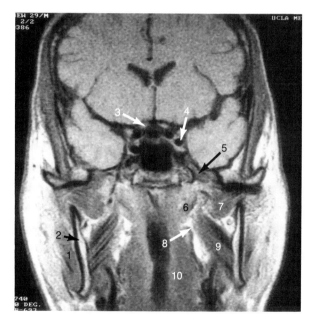

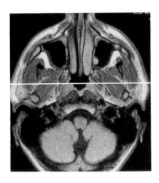

1, lateral pterygoid
   muscle
2, optic nerve
3, sphenoid sinus
4, inferior orbital fissure
5, zygomatic arch
6, fossa of Rosenmueller
7, torus tubarius
8, eustachian tube
9, nasopharynx
10, parapharyngeal space
11, masseter muscle
12, medial pterygoid
    muscle

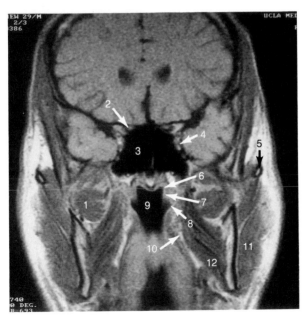

1, medial pterygoid muscle
2, lateral pterygoid muscle
3, temporalis muscle
4, optic nerve
5, sphenoid sinus
6, zygomatic arch
7, nasopharynx
8, mandible
9, masseter muscle

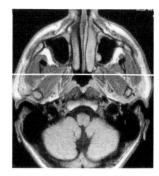

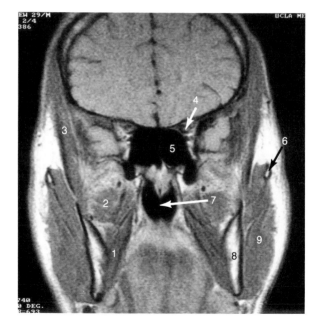

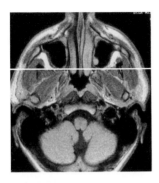

1, mandible
2, medial pterygoid muscle
3, pterygopalatine fossa
4, optic nerve
5, nasal septum
6, sphenoid sinus
7, temporalis muscle
8, middle turbinate
9, zygomatic arch
10, inferior turbinate
11, masseter muscle

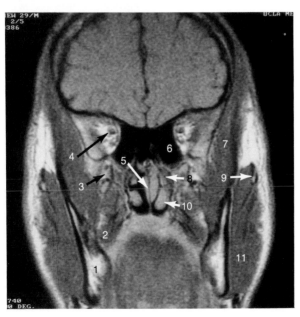

1, lateral rectus muscle
2, optic nerve
3, medial rectus muscle
4, superior oblique
   muscle
5, ethmoid sinuses
6, superior rectus muscle
7, superior ophthalmic
   vein
8, inferior rectus muscle
9, middle turbinate
10, maxillary sinus
11, inferior turbinate

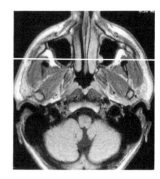

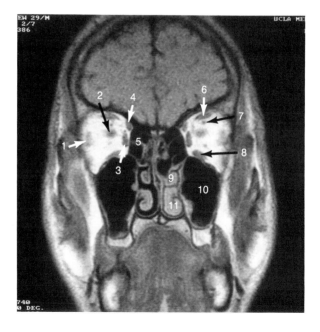

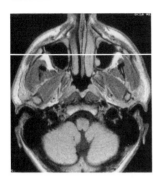

1, inferior turbinate
2, middle turbinate
3, globe
4, superior oblique muscle
5, ethmoid sinus
6, medial rectus muscle
7, frontal sinus
8, superior ophthalmic vein
9, superior rectus muscle
10, lateral rectus muscle
11, inferior rectus muscle
12, maxillary sinus
13, teeth

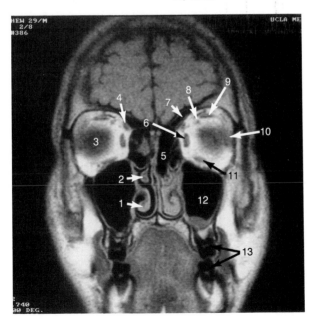

1, lateral rectus muscle
2, globe
3, frontal sinus
4, crista galli
5, ethmoid sinus
6, superior ophthalmic vein
7, superior oblique muscle
8, superior rectus muscle
9, medial rectus muscle
10, inferior oblique muscle
11, middle turbinate
12, maxillary sinus
13, inferior turbinate

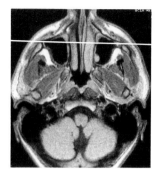

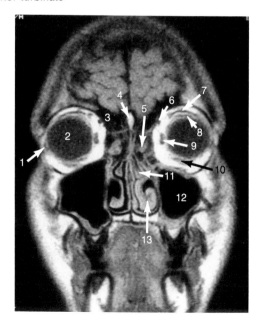

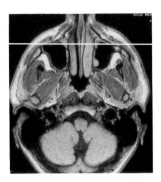

1, frontal sinus
2, ethmoid sinus
3, superior ophthalmic
   vein
4, globe
5, middle turbinate
6, maxillary sinus
7, inferior turbinate
8, hard palate

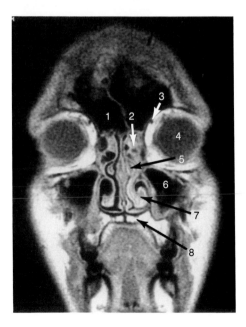

1, frontal sinus
2, nasal vault
3, ethmoid sinus
4, nasal septum
5, maxillary sinus
6, inferior turbinates
7, hard palate

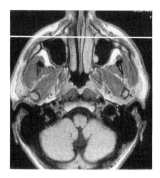

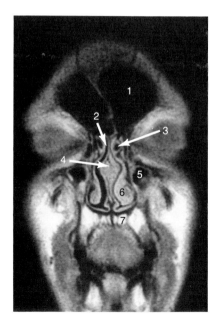

Temporal Bone _____

1, masseter muscle
2, lateral pterygoid muscle
3, mandible
4, facial nerve
5, hypoglossal canal
6, mastoid air cells

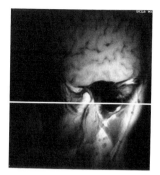

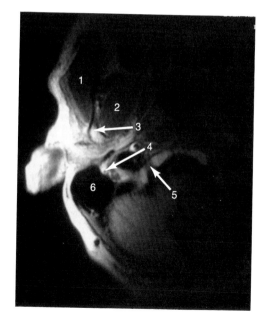

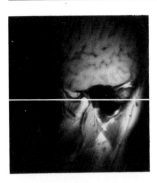

1, external auditory canal
2, mandibular condyle
3, clivus
4, carotid artery
5, cranial nerves IX–XI
6, jugular foramen
7, facial nerve
8, mastoid air cells

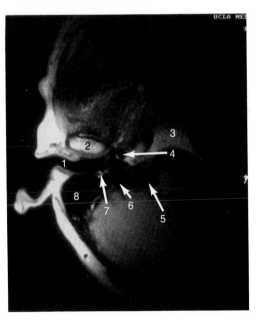

1, mastoid air cells
2, temporomandibular
   joint
3, clivus
4, carotid artery
5, facial nerve
6, flocculus of cerebellum

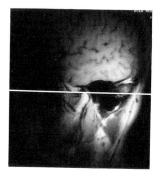

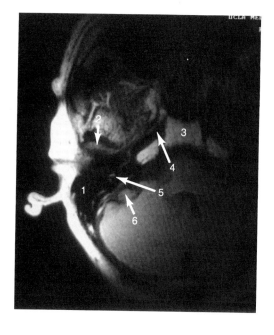

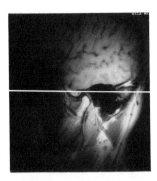

1, flocculus of cerebellum
2, mastoid air cells
3, vestibule
4, cochlea
5, temporal lobe
6, internal carotid artery
7, internal auditory canal
8, sphenoid sinus

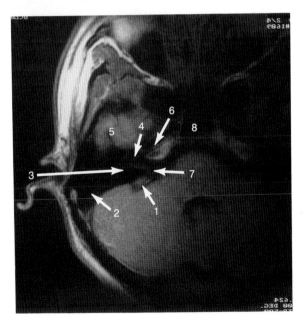

1, temporal lobe
2, petrous ridge
3, carotid artery

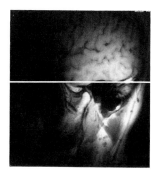

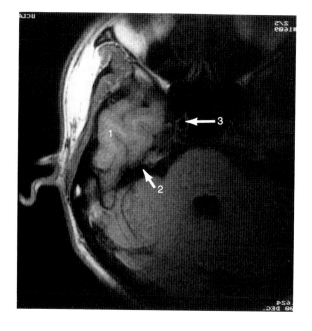

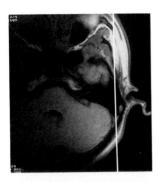

1, temporal lobe
2, condyle
3, external auditory canal
4, mastoid air cells

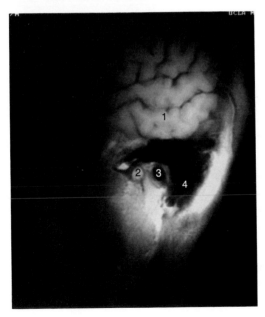

1, temporomandibular joint
2, temporal lobe
3, cerebellum
4, sigmoid sinus
5, mastoid air cells
6, facial nerve
7, condyle

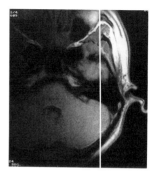

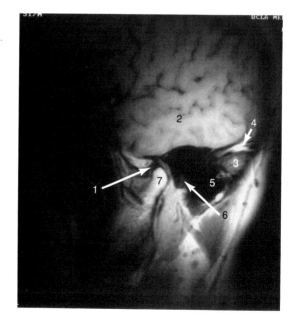

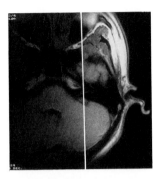

1, temporal lobe
2, internal carotid artery
3, internal auditory canal
4, cerebellum

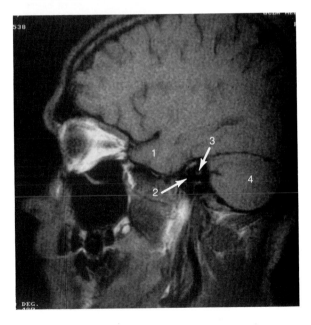

1, temporal lobe
2, intratemporal facial nerve
3, stylomastoid foramen
4, mastoid air cells

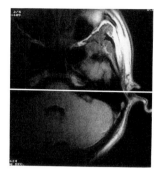

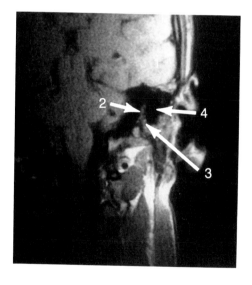

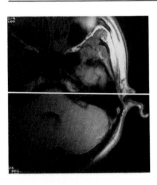

1, cochlear nerve
2, facial nerve
3, temporal lobe
4, external auditory canal
5, jugular vein

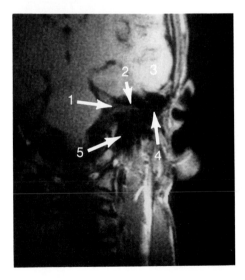

1, temporal lobe
2, external auditory canal
3, parotid gland
4, internal carotid artery

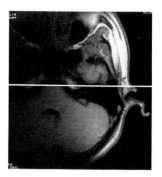

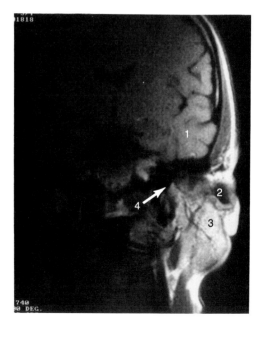

References

1. Lufkin RB, Larsson S, Hanafee W. NMR anatomy of the larynx and tongue base. *Radiology* 1983; 148(1):173–175.

2. Lufkin RB, Hanafee WN. Application of surface coils to MR anatomy of the larynx. *Am J Neuroradiol* 1985;6:491–497.

3. Lufkin RB, Hanafee WN, Wortham D, et al. Larynx and hypopharynx: MR imaging with surface coils. *Radiology* 1986;158(3):747–754.

4. Lufkin RB, Wortham DG, Dietrich RB, et al. Tongue and oropharynx: findings on MR imaging. *Radiology* 1986;161:69–75.

5. Dietrich R, Lufkin R, Kangarloo H, et al. Head and neck MR imaging in pediatric patient. *Radiology* 1986;159:769–776.

6. Teresi L, Lufkin R, Wortham D, et al. MRI of the normal intratemporal facial nerve. *Am J Neuroradiol* 1987;8:44–49.

7. Teresi L, Lufkin R, Kolin E, et al. MRI of the intra-parotid facial nerve. *Am J Roentgenol* 1987;148(5):995–1000.

8. Teresi L, Lufkin R, Wortham D, et al. Parotid masses: magnetic resonance imaging. *Radiology* 1987;163(2):405–411.

9. Teresi LM, Lufkin RB, Vinuela F, et al. MR imaging of the nasopharynx and floor of the middle cranial fossa. I. Normal anatomy. *Radiology* 1987;164(3): 811–816.

10. Christianson R, Lufkin R, Hanafee W. MRI of the mandible. *Radiology (in press)*.